RYAN STONE

Colon Cancer Prevention and Management

A Comprehensive Guide to Diet and Nutrition

Contents

1

INTRODUCTION

Millions of people throughout the world suffer from the terrible illness known as colon cancer. Colon cancer is the third most prevalent cancer diagnosis and the third highest cause of cancer deaths in the United States, according to the American Cancer Society. While there are several risk factors that can lead to colon cancer, diet and lifestyle decisions are extremely important in preventing and managing the disease.

This in-depth manual will cover the connection between diet and colon cancer, the significance of a healthy diet during treatment, and lifestyle variables that affect colon health. We will give you helpful pointers and recommendations to assist you in making easy but effective dietary and lifestyle adjustments to enhance the health of your colon and lower your risk of colon cancer.

CHAPTER ONE

UNDERSTANDING COLON CANCER

ypes of colon cancer

1.Adenocarcinoma: Making up around 96% of all occurrences of colon cancer, this is the most prevalent kind. Adenocarcinomas can appear anywhere in the colon and rectum and grow in the glandular cells that line the interior of these organs.

2.Carcinoid tumors: These are uncommon, slowly growing tumors that often appear in the rectum and colon, which are parts of the digestive tract. They develop from neuroendocrine cells and have the capacity to create hormones that result in symptoms like flushing and diarrhea.

3.Gastrointestinal stromal tumors (GISTs): are uncommon

tumors that develop in the colon and rectum's muscle or connective tissue. Although GISTs are typically benign, some can develop into malignancy.

4.Lymphoma: This uncommon kind of cancer develops in the rectum and colon's lymphatic tissue. Although lymphoma can affect persons of any age, it is most prevalent in those over 60.

5.Sarcoma: This uncommon kind of cancer appears in the muscle and fat layers as well as the connective tissue of the colon and rectum. Less than 1% of all colon malignancies are sarcomas.

Getting a correct diagnosis is essential to receiving appropriate therapy since different kinds of colon cancer may require various therapeutic modalities and result in various clinical outcomes. Regular screening exams can aid in the early detection of colon cancer, when it is most curable.

Risk factors for colon cancer

1.Age: People over 50 are more likely to develop colon cancer. Most cases are detected in adults over 60, and the risk rises with age.

2.Personal or family history of colon cancer: You are more likely to have the disease if you or a close relative has had it or certain types of polyps.

3.IBD: Colon cancer risk is higher in those with ulcerative colitis or Crohn's disease than in people without these illnesses.

4.Genetics: Certain hereditary gene mutations, such as Lynch syndrome and familial adenomatous polyposis (FAP), can raise the risk of developing colon cancer.

5.Lifestyle factors: Certain lifestyle practices, such as a diet high in red and processed meat, inactivity, obesity, smoking, and heavy alcohol consumption, can raise the risk of colon cancer.

6.Type 2 diabetes: Insulin resistance and inflammation may contribute to the increased risk of colon cancer in people with type 2 diabetes.

African Americans and Jews of Eastern European heritage (Ashkenazi Jews) have the highest rates of colon cancer in the United States, respectively.

There are things you can do to lower your risk even while some risk factors, like age and genetics, cannot be changed. Keeping a healthy weight, engaging in regular exercise, and quitting smoking can all help reduce your risk of colon cancer.

Symptoms of colon cancer

1.Bowel habits: Constipation, diarrhea, or changes in the regularity or consistency of bowel motions can all be symptoms of colon cancer.

2.Rectal bleeding or blood in the stool: Colon cancer is one illness that might show symptoms of blood in the stool. It could be black and tarry or bright red.

3.Constant stomach discomfort or cramping may be an indication of colon cancer, particularly if it coexists with other symptoms.

4.Weakness or anemia: Anemia, or having too few red blood cells, can make you feel weak or anemia. A continuous hemorrhage from colon cancer can result in anemia.

5.Unintentional weight loss: Losing weight without attempting to may be a symptom of colon cancer among other illnesses.

6.Narrow stools: If your stools start to get narrower than usual, this may indicate a colon obstruction.

7.Bloating or fullness: Even after consuming only a small amount of food, colon cancer might result in a sense of bloating or fullness.

It's crucial to remember that a lot of these symptoms can also be brought on by other, less severe diseases. However, it's crucial to speak with your healthcare provider if you are suffering any of these symptoms, especially if they last more than a few days, to ascertain the cause and the best course of action. Additionally, regular colon cancer screenings can aid in the early detection of the disease.

Stages of colon cancer

The earliest stage of colon cancer is known as stage 0 or carcinoma in situ. The cancer cells have not moved to other tissues and are exclusively present in the deepest layer of the colon or rectum.

Stage I: At this point, the cancer has only penetrated a portion of the colon or rectum's deeper layers and has not yet spread outside.

Stage II: At this point, the cancer may have invaded neigh-boring tissues and broken through the colon or rectum's wall, but it has not yet spread to any close lymph nodes or distant organs.

Stage III: At this point, the cancer has not yet progressed to distant organs but has spread to adjacent lymph nodes.

Stage IV: At this point, the cancer has spread to adjacent lymph nodes as well as distant organs like the liver or lungs.

It's crucial to understand that a number of variables, including the size and location of the tumor, its invasion depth into the colon or rectum, whether it has spread to surrounding lymph nodes, and whether it has reached distant organs, determine the stage of colon cancer. The stage of colon cancer is crucial for selecting the right treatment strategy and forecasting results.

Screening and diagnosis of colon cancer

Screening:

Colonoscopy:The most common screening procedure for colon cancer is a colonoscopy. A flexible tube with a camera on the end is advanced down the colon during a colonoscopy to check for any abnormalities, such as polyps or tumors.

Test for fecal occult blood: This procedure looks for blood in the stool, which may be a symptom of colon cancer. It is a simple test that you may perform at home.

Stool DNA test: This test scans the stool for particular DNA traces that may point to the existence of precancerous polyps or colon cancer.

Diagnosis:

Biopsy: A biopsy may be performed to remove a tiny sample of tissue for microscopic inspection if abnormalities are discovered during a colonoscopy or other screening test.

Imaging tests: Imaging tests, such as CT scans, MRIs, or PET scans, can be used to detect the presence of colon cancer or to assess its severity.

Blood tests: Blood tests, including the carcinoembryonic antigen (CEA) test, can be used to track blood levels of specific proteins that may be raised in persons with colon cancer.

Additional tests might be performed if colon cancer is found to ascertain the cancer's stage and whether it has spread to other body parts. This data forecasts outcomes and aids in treatment decision-making. Depending on the stage and severity of the illness, treatment options for colon cancer may include surgery, radiation therapy, chemotherapy, targeted therapy, or immunotherapy.

3

CHAPTER TWO

THE ROLE OF DIET IN COLON CANCER PREVENTION AND MANAGEMENT

The link between diet and colon cancer

It is thought that diet has a big impact on colon cancer development. A higher risk of colon cancer has been linked to a number of dietary factors, including:

Meats that are red and processed, such as beef, pig, and hot dogs, in excessive quantities have been associated to an increased risk of colon cancer. These meats include substances that can irritate the gut lining and exacerbate inflammation.

Diets heavy in saturated and trans fats, which are present in fried foods, processed snacks, and baked products, have been associated with an elevated risk of colon cancer.

A diet deficient in fiber, especially from fruits, vegetables, and whole grains, has been associated with an elevated risk of colon cancer. Fiber helps to maintain a healthy digestive system and can assist to lessen colon inflammation.

Alcohol consumption: Excessive alcohol drinking has been associated with a higher risk of colon cancer.

However, some dietary elements, such as the following, may help lower the risk of colon cancer:

Consuming a diet rich in fiber from fruits, vegetables, and whole grains may help lower the chance of developing colon cancer.

Calcium consumption: According to studies, having enough calcium in your diet may help lower your chance of developing colon cancer.

Diet that is primarily composed of plants: A vegetarian or Mediterranean-style diet that is mostly composed of plants may help lower the risk of colon cancer.

Overall, consuming less red and processed meat, saturated and trans fats, and alcohol while keeping a healthy and balanced diet that includes lots of fruits, vegetables, whole grains, and lean protein sources may help lower the risk of colon cancer.

The benefits of a healthy diet for colon health

Lowers risk of colon cancer: A diet rich in fiber, fruits, vegetables, and whole grains can help lessen the risk of colon inflammation.

Encourages regular bowel movements: Eating a fiber-rich diet helps maintain a healthy digestive tract and encourages regular bowel movements, which can lower the chance of developing colon cancer.

supports a healthy gut microbiome: The colon's microbial population, known as the gut microbiome, is crucial to colon health. A healthy gut flora can promote a diet rich in fiber and plant-based foods, which may help lower the risk of colon cancer.

Provides essential nutrients: Essential nutrients, such as vitamins, minerals, and antioxidants, are crucial for overall health and can help lower the chance of developing colon cancer. These nutrients are found in a balanced diet that includes a range of fruits, vegetables, and lean protein sources.

Promotes weight management: By eating a balanced diet and doing regular exercise, one can help lower their risk of acquiring colon cancer.

Overall, eating a balanced diet that emphasizes fresh produce, whole grains, lean protein sources, and avoiding red and processed meats, saturated and trans fats, and alcohol can have a positive impact on colon health and lower the chance of getting colon cancer.

Foods to eat and avoid for colon cancer prevention

Foods to Eat to Prevent Colon Cancer:

1.Foods High in Fiber: Eating a fiber-rich diet can help lower the risk of colon cancer. Whole grains, produce, fruits, vegetables, beans, and nuts are all excellent sources of fiber.

2.Fruits and vegetables:Fruits and vegetables are a good source of vitamins, minerals, and antioxidants that are beneficial to overall health and can lower the risk of colon cancer. To receive a diversity of nutrients, try to eat a variety of colored fruits and vegetables.

3.Fish: Consuming fish, especially fatty fish high in omega-3 fatty acids like salmon, tuna, and mackerel, can help reduce inflammation in the body and may lessen the risk of colon cancer.

4.Probiotic Foods: Probiotic foods can aid in maintaining a healthy gut microbiome, which is crucial for colon health. Examples of probiotic foods include yogurt, kefir, sauerkraut, and kimchi.

5.Foods High in Calcium: Consuming adequate calcium daily may lower the risk of developing colon cancer. Leafy greens, dairy products, and fortified foods are all excellent sources of calcium.

Foods to Avoid to Prevent Colon Cancer:

1.Red and processed meat:Meats that are red and processed, such as beef, pig, and hot dogs, in excessive quantities have been associated to an increased risk of colon cancer. These meats include substances that can irritate the gut lining and exacerbate inflammation.

2.Saturated and Trans Fats: Colon cancer risk has been linked to diets high in saturated and trans fats, which are included in fried foods, processed snacks, and baked products.

3.Drinks with added sugar: Regular consumption of drinks with added sugar, such as soda and fruit juice, has been associated to an increased risk of colon cancer.

4.Alcohol: Excessive alcohol consumption has been associated with a higher risk of colon cancer.

5.Refined Grains: Consuming a diet high in refined grains, such as white rice, pasta, and bread, has been associated with a higher risk of colon cancer. Choose whole grain alternatives instead.

A diet low in red and processed meats, saturated and trans fats, sugar-sweetened beverages, alcohol, and refined grains and high in fiber, fruits, vegetables, and omega-3 fatty acids can help lower the risk of colon cancer.

How diet can support colon cancer treatment

Nutritional Balance: It's crucial to keep your food healthy and balanced while you're receiving treatment for colon cancer. To boost the immune system and help the body deal with the adverse effects of therapy, it's important to make sure the body gets enough protein, healthy fats, complex carbs, vitamins, and minerals.

Managing Adverse Reactions: Several adverse effects of colon cancer treatment, such as nausea, vomiting, diarrhea, constipation, and loss of appetite, are possible. You can get advice on how to manage these side effects through food from a trained dietitian. For instance, eating easily digestible, short, frequent meals can reduce nausea and vomiting. Drinking enough of liquids can help stop the dehydration that diarrhea can cause. Constipation can be relieved by consuming high-fiber foods and drinking plenty of fluids.

Immune system booster: Consuming a diet high in nutrients, such as fruits, vegetables, whole grains, lean protein, and healthy fats, can support the body's capacity to fight cancer and strengthen the immune system.

Reducing Inflammation: One typical adverse effect of colon cancer treatment is inflammation. Consuming a diet high in anti-inflammatory foods, such as fatty fish, olive oil, nuts, seeds, fruits, and vegetables, can aid in reducing inflammation and promoting the body's capacity to heal.

Managing Weight: The therapy for colon cancer might result in weight reduction, weight gain, or swings in weight. A balanced diet and regular exercise can help patients achieve better treatment results and lower their risk of cancer recurrence.

Avoiding Specific Foods: It's critical to stay away from specific items that can complicate or obstruct treatment when receiving treatment for colon cancer. While grapefruit and its juice might hinder the absorption of some drugs, raw or undercooked meat, seafood, and eggs can raise the risk of infection.

Overall, adopting a nutritious, well-balanced diet high in foods that reduce inflammation and good fats can support colon cancer treatment and enhance treatment results. By collaborating with a certified dietitian, you can make sure that your nutritional requirements are satisfied and that you can effectively manage any adverse effects of your treatment through diet.

4

CHAPTER THREE

THE POWER OF FIBER FOR COLON HEALTH

hat is fiber and why is it important for colon health

Fiber is a type of carbohydrate that is found in plant-based foods, such as fruits, vegetables, whole grains, nuts, and seeds. It is an essential nutrient that plays a crucial role in maintaining colon health.

There are two types of fiber: soluble fiber and insoluble fiber. Soluble fiber dissolves in water and forms a gel-like substance in the intestines, while insoluble fiber does not dissolve in water and adds bulk to the stool. Both types of fiber are important for colon health.

Fiber is important for colon health for several reasons:

Promotes Regular Bowel Movements: Fiber helps promote regular bowel movements by adding bulk to the stool, which helps move waste through the intestines. This can help prevent constipation, which can lead to the development of hemorrhoids and other digestive disorders.

Prevents Diverticulosis: Diverticulosis is a condition in which small pockets form in the colon wall, which can become inflamed and infected. A diet high in fiber can help prevent diverticulosis by promoting regular bowel movements and reducing pressure on the colon wall.

Reduces the Risk of Colon Cancer: Studies have shown that a diet high in fiber can reduce the risk of colon cancer. Fiber helps remove waste and toxins from the colon, which can reduce the risk of cancer-causing agents coming into contact with the colon wall.

Controls Blood Sugar: Fiber can help control blood sugar levels by slowing down the absorption of sugar into the bloodstream. This can help prevent spikes and crashes in blood sugar levels, which can lead to the development of diabetes and other health problems.

Promotes Weight Loss: Fiber can help promote weight loss by adding bulk to the diet, which can help increase feelings of fullness and reduce overall calorie intake. This can help reduce the risk of obesity, which is a risk factor for colon cancer.

The recommended daily intake of fiber is 25 grams for women and 38 grams for men. However, most people do not consume enough fiber in their diets. To increase fiber intake, it is recommended to eat a variety of fiber-rich foods, such as fruits, vegetables, whole grains, nuts, and seeds. It is also important to drink plenty of water to help the fiber move through the digestive system. A diet high in fiber can help promote colon health and reduce the risk of colon cancer and other digestive disorders.

Types of fiber and their benefits

As mentioned previously, there are two types of fiber: soluble and insoluble. While both types of fiber are important for overall health, they have different benefits for the body.

1.Soluble Fiber: Soluble fiber dissolves in water and forms a gel-like substance in the intestines. This type of fiber is found in foods such as oats, beans, peas, apples, and carrots. The benefits of soluble fiber include:

Lowering Cholesterol: Soluble fiber can help lower LDL (bad) cholesterol levels by binding to cholesterol in the intestines and preventing it from being absorbed into the bloodstream.

Regulating Blood Sugar: Soluble fiber can help regulate blood sugar levels by slowing down the absorption of sugar into the bloodstream. This can help prevent spikes and crashes in blood sugar levels, which can lead to the development of diabetes and other health problems.

Promoting Feelings of Fullness: Soluble fiber can help promote feelings of fullness, which can help reduce overall calorie intake and promote weight loss.

2.Insoluble Fiber: Insoluble fiber does not dissolve in water and adds bulk to the stool. This type of fiber is found in foods such as wheat bran, nuts, and many vegetables. The benefits of insoluble fiber include:

Promoting Regular Bowel Movements: Insoluble fiber adds bulk to the stool, which can help move waste through the intestines and promote regular bowel movements. This can help prevent constipation and other digestive disorders.

Preventing Diverticulosis: Insoluble fiber can help prevent diverticulosis by promoting regular bowel movements and reducing pressure on the colon wall.

Reducing the Risk of Colon Cancer: Insoluble fiber can help reduce the risk of colon cancer by promoting regular bowel movements and reducing the amount of time waste stays in the colon.

It is important to note that many foods contain both soluble and insoluble fiber. For example, whole grains such as oats and barley contain both types of fiber. It is recommended to consume a variety of fiber-rich foods to get the full range of benefits that both types of fiber offer.

Both types of fiber are important for overall health and should be included in a healthy diet. Soluble fiber can help lower cholesterol, regulate blood sugar, and promote feelings of fullness, while insoluble fiber can promote regular bowel movements, prevent diverticulosis, and reduce the risk of colon cancer.

How much fiber should you eat for colon health

The amount of fiber recommended for optimal colon health

depends on several factors, such as age, sex, and physical activity level. The Institute of Medicine (IOM) provides dietary guidelines for fiber intake based on age and sex. The recommended daily intake of fiber for adults under the age of 50 is 25 grams for women and 38 grams for men. For adults over the age of 50, the recommended daily intake decreases to 21 grams for women and 30 grams for men.

It is important to note that these recommendations are based on the average daily intake needed to maintain overall health, not specifically for colon health. However, studies have shown that increasing fiber intake can help prevent colon cancer and other digestive disorders.

For individuals who are not currently meeting the recommended daily intake of fiber, it is important to increase fiber intake gradually to avoid digestive discomfort such as bloating, gas, and abdominal pain. It is also important to consume adequate amounts of water to prevent constipation and promote regular bowel movements.

It is recommended to consume a variety of fiber-rich foods such as whole grains, fruits, vegetables, nuts, and legumes to obtain the full range of health benefits. Some examples of high-fiber foods include:

Whole grain bread and cereals
  Brown rice
  Quinoa
  Fruits such as apples, berries, and oranges
  Vegetables such as broccoli, spinach, and carrots

Nuts and seeds such as almonds, chia seeds, and flaxseeds

Legumes such as lentils, black beans, and chickpeas

The recommended daily intake of fiber for adults varies based on age and sex, but increasing fiber intake can help promote colon health and reduce the risk of colon cancer and other digestive disorders. It is important to increase fiber intake gradually and consume a variety of fiber-rich foods to obtain the full range of health benefits.

Fiber-rich foods to add to your diet

Fiber-rich foods should be a staple in any healthy diet, as they provide a range of health benefits including promoting colon health, regulating blood sugar, reducing cholesterol levels, and maintaining a healthy weight. Here are some fiber-rich foods to consider adding to your diet:

1.Whole grains: Whole grains such as oats, barley, brown rice, quinoa, and whole wheat bread are high in fiber and provide long-lasting energy. They also contain essential nutrients such as B vitamins, iron, and magnesium.

2.Fruits: Many fruits are high in fiber, particularly when consumed with the skin intact. Apples, pears, berries, oranges, and kiwis are all great options. Additionally, fruits are a good source of vitamins and antioxidants, which can help prevent chronic diseases.

3.Vegetables: Vegetables are a great source of fiber and should be a staple in any healthy diet. Broccoli, carrots, kale, spinach, and Brussels sprouts are particularly high in fiber. They are also rich in essential vitamins, minerals, and antioxidants.

4.Legumes: Legumes such as lentils, beans, and chickpeas are excellent sources of fiber and protein. They are also a good source of iron, potassium, and folate. Incorporating legumes into your diet can help improve digestion and promote heart health.

5.Nuts and seeds: Nuts and seeds are a great source of healthy fats, protein, and fiber. Almonds, chia seeds, flaxseeds, and pumpkin seeds are particularly high in fiber. They also contain essential vitamins and minerals such as vitamin E, magnesium, and zinc.

6.High-fiber snacks: Snacking on fiber-rich foods can help promote satiety and prevent overeating. Some great options include popcorn, whole grain crackers, and sliced vegetables with hummus or nut butter.

Incorporating these fiber-rich foods into your diet can help promote overall health and wellbeing. It is important to gradually increase fiber intake to avoid digestive discomfort and to drink plenty of water to support digestion. Additionally, it is recommended to consume a variety of fiber-rich foods to obtain the full range of health benefits.

5

CHAPTER FOUR

EATING TO REDUCE INFLAMMATION AND BOOST IMMUNITY

T*he connection between inflammation, immunity, and colon cancer*

Inflammation is a natural response of the immune system to injury or infection. It is an essential process that helps to remove damaged tissue, fight off infections, and promote tissue repair. However, chronic inflammation can be harmful to the body and has been linked to the development of several chronic diseases, including colon cancer.

Inflammation can play a role in the development of colon cancer in several ways. Firstly, chronic inflammation can damage the DNA in colon cells, leading to mutations that can trigger the development of cancerous cells. Secondly, inflammation can promote the growth and survival of cancer cells by creating an environment that supports their growth and proliferation. Finally, inflammation can also suppress the immune system, which is an essential defense against cancer development.

The immune system plays a critical role in protecting the body against cancer. It is responsible for detecting and destroying cancer cells before they can develop into tumors. However, chronic inflammation can weaken the immune system, making it less effective at detecting and destroying cancer cells. In addition, chronic inflammation can also promote the growth and proliferation of immune cells that promote the development of cancer.

Several factors can contribute to chronic inflammation in the body, including a poor diet, stress, lack of exercise, and exposure to environmental toxins. A diet that is high in processed foods, sugar, and unhealthy fats can promote inflammation in the body, while a diet rich in anti-inflammatory foods can help to reduce inflammation and support immune function.

Some of the best anti-inflammatory foods for colon health include fruits and vegetables, whole grains, nuts, seeds, and fatty fish. These foods are rich in antioxidants and anti-inflammatory compounds that can help to reduce inflammation in the body and support immune function. In addition, it is important to limit your intake of processed foods, sugar, and unhealthy fats, as these foods can promote inflammation in the body.

In summary, chronic inflammation can play a significant role in the development of colon cancer by damaging DNA, promoting the growth and survival of cancer cells, and suppressing immune function. A diet that is rich in anti-inflammatory foods and low in processed foods, sugar, and unhealthy fats can help to reduce inflammation in the body and support immune function, which can help to reduce the risk of colon cancer development.

Anti-inflammatory foods for colon health

Inflammation is a natural response of the immune system to injury or infection. However, chronic inflammation can contribute to the development of several chronic diseases, including colon cancer. An anti-inflammatory diet can help to reduce inflammation in the body and support immune function, which can help to reduce the risk of colon cancer development.

Here are some of the best anti-inflammatory foods for colon health:

1.Fruits and Vegetables: Fruits and vegetables are rich in antioxidants and anti-inflammatory compounds that can help to reduce inflammation in the body. Some of the best fruits and vegetables for colon health include leafy greens, berries, citrus fruits, tomatoes, and cruciferous vegetables like broccoli and cauliflower.

2.Whole Grains: Whole grains are a rich source of fiber, which can help to promote regular bowel movements and reduce the risk of colon cancer. Some of the best whole grains for colon health include oats, brown rice, quinoa, and barley.

3.Nuts and Seeds: Nuts and seeds are rich in healthy fats

and anti-inflammatory compounds that can help to reduce inflammation in the body. Some of the best nuts and seeds for colon health include almonds, walnuts, chia seeds, and flaxseeds.

4.Fatty Fish: Fatty fish like salmon, tuna, and sardines are rich in omega-3 fatty acids, which have been shown to have anti-inflammatory effects in the body. These fatty acids can also help to promote immune function and reduce the risk of colon cancer development.

5.Herbs and Spices: Herbs and spices are a rich source of anti-inflammatory compounds that can help to reduce inflammation in the body. Some of the best herbs and spices for colon health include ginger, turmeric, garlic, and cinnamon.

In addition to these foods, it is important to limit your intake of processed foods, sugar, and unhealthy fats, as these foods can promote inflammation in the body. By incorporating more anti-inflammatory foods into your diet and limiting your intake of inflammatory foods, you can help to reduce inflammation in the body and support immune function, which can help to reduce the risk of colon cancer development.

Immune-boosting foods for colon health

The immune system plays a critical role in protecting the body from infections and diseases, including colon cancer. By incorporating immune-boosting foods into your diet, you can help to support immune function and reduce the risk of colon cancer development. Here are some of the best immune-boosting foods for colon health:

Citrus Fruits: Citrus fruits like oranges, lemons, and grapefruits are rich in vitamin C, which is a powerful antioxidant that can help to support immune function. Vitamin C can also help to reduce inflammation in the body and promote healthy digestion, which can reduce the risk of colon cancer.

Leafy Greens: Leafy greens like spinach, kale, and Swiss chard are rich in antioxidants and anti-inflammatory compounds that can help to support immune function. These greens are also rich in fiber, which can help to promote healthy digestion and reduce the risk of colon cancer.

Berries: Berries like blueberries, raspberries, and strawberries are rich in antioxidants and polyphenols, which have been shown to have immune-boosting effects. These compounds can also help to reduce inflammation in the body and protect against the development of colon cancer.

Garlic: Garlic is a rich source of sulfur compounds, which have been shown to have immune-boosting effects. These compounds can also help to reduce inflammation in the body and protect against the development of colon cancer.

Yogurt: Yogurt is rich in probiotics, which are beneficial bacteria that can help to support immune function and promote healthy digestion. Probiotics can also help to reduce inflammation in the body and reduce the risk of colon cancer.

Mushrooms: Mushrooms like shiitake, maitake, and reishi are rich in beta-glucans, which have been shown to have immune-boosting effects. These compounds can also help to reduce inflammation in the body and protect against the development of colon cancer.

In addition to these foods, it is important to eat a well-balanced diet that includes plenty of fruits, vegetables, whole grains, and lean protein sources. It is also important to limit your intake of processed foods, sugar, and unhealthy fats, which can promote inflammation in the body and reduce immune function. By incorporating immune-boosting foods into your diet and limiting your intake of inflammatory foods, you can help to support immune function and reduce the risk of colon cancer development.

Recipes that feature these ingredients

Here are some delicious recipes that feature the immune-boosting foods for colon health:

1.Citrus and Kale Salad: This refreshing salad is packed with immune-boosting nutrients from citrus fruits and kale. To make it, simply chop up some kale and mix it with orange and grapefruit segments. Top with a simple vinaigrette made from olive oil, apple cider vinegar, honey, and Dijon mustard.

2.Mixed Berry Smoothie: This smoothie is a delicious way to incorporate immune-boosting berries into your diet. Simply blend together a cup of mixed berries (such as blueberries, raspberries, and strawberries), a banana, and some almond milk. For an extra boost, add a spoonful of chia seeds or flaxseed meal.

3.Garlic Roasted Vegetables: Roasted vegetables are a delicious and easy way to incorporate immune-boosting garlic into your diet. To make them, simply chop up your favorite vegetables (such as carrots, broccoli, and cauliflower) and toss them with olive oil and minced garlic. Roast in the oven until tender and crispy.

4.Yogurt Parfait: This simple and tasty breakfast or snack is a great way to incorporate immune-boosting yogurt into your diet. Simply layer Greek yogurt with your favorite fruits (such as berries or sliced bananas) and granola. For an extra boost, top with a spoonful of honey or chopped nuts.

5.Mushroom and Spinach Omelet: This savory omelet is a delicious way to incorporate immune-boosting mushrooms and leafy greens into your diet. To make it, sauté some sliced mushrooms and spinach in a pan until tender. Beat a few eggs and pour them over the vegetables. Cook until set, then fold over and serve.

By incorporating these immune-boosting foods into your diet, you can support immune function and reduce the risk of colon cancer development. Try out these recipes and experiment with other ways to incorporate these ingredients into your meals for a delicious and healthy diet.

6

CHAPTER FIVE

NUTRITION DURING COLON CANCER TREATMENT

he importance of good nutrition during colon cancer treatment

Good nutrition is essential during colon cancer treatment to help manage symptoms, maintain strength and energy, and support the body's healing process. Cancer treatment can often cause side effects that impact the digestive system and make it difficult to eat, including nausea, vomiting, diarrhea, constipation, and loss of appetite. In addition, chemotherapy and radiation therapy can damage healthy cells and tissues, making it important to nourish the body with the right nutrients to support healing and recovery.

Here are some ways that good nutrition can help during colon cancer treatment:

Manage side effects: Certain foods can help manage side effects of colon cancer treatment. For example, ginger can help alleviate nausea and vomiting, while high-fiber foods can help prevent constipation. Drinking plenty of fluids can also help prevent dehydration and promote regular bowel movements.

Maintain energy and strength: Eating a balanced diet with plenty of protein, complex carbohydrates, and healthy fats can help maintain energy levels and prevent muscle wasting. Foods high in protein, such as lean meats, fish, poultry, and legumes, can help build and repair tissues and promote healing.

Boost immunity: A diet rich in immune-boosting nutrients, such as vitamin C, vitamin E, and zinc, can help support the body's immune system and promote healing. Eating a variety of fruits, vegetables, whole grains, and lean proteins can help ensure that the body gets all the essential nutrients it needs.

Support healing: Certain nutrients, such as antioxidants and omega-3 fatty acids, can help reduce inflammation and promote healing. Foods high in antioxidants, such as berries, leafy greens, and nuts, can help protect healthy cells from damage, while foods high in omega-3s, such as fatty fish, can help reduce inflammation and promote heart health.

During colon cancer treatment, it is important to work with a registered dietitian to develop an individualized nutrition plan that meets your unique needs and preferences. A dietitian can help you identify foods that may help manage side effects, provide tips for meal planning and preparation, and ensure that your diet provides all the necessary nutrients to support healing and recovery. With the right nutrition plan, you can support your body during colon cancer treatment and improve your overall quality of life.

Common side effects that affect diet and nutrition

Colon cancer treatment can cause a range of side effects that can impact diet and nutrition. These side effects can vary depending on the type of treatment and the individual's overall health, but here are some of the most common ones:

Nausea and vomiting: Nausea and vomiting are common side effects of chemotherapy and radiation therapy. These symptoms can make it difficult to eat and drink, leading to dehydration and malnutrition. Eating small, frequent meals throughout the day and avoiding strong-smelling or greasy foods may help manage nausea.

Diarrhea and constipation: Colon cancer treatment can also cause changes in bowel movements, including diarrhea and constipation. Diarrhea can lead to dehydration and electrolyte imbalances, while constipation can cause discomfort and bloating. Eating foods high in fiber, such as fruits, vegetables, and whole grains, can help prevent constipation, while avoiding foods that can irritate the digestive system, such as caffeine and spicy foods, can help manage diarrhea.

Loss of appetite: Cancer treatment can cause a loss of appetite, which can lead to malnutrition and weight loss. Eating small, frequent meals and choosing nutrient-dense foods can help ensure that the body gets the necessary nutrients, even if the appetite is low.

Taste changes: Chemotherapy can cause changes in taste, making foods taste metallic or bland. This can lead to a decreased desire to eat and can make it difficult to consume nutrient-rich foods. Trying different flavors and textures, using herbs and spices to add flavor, and avoiding strong-smelling or flavored foods may help manage taste changes.

Fatigue: Colon cancer treatment can cause fatigue, which can make it difficult to prepare meals or eat a balanced diet. Eating small, frequent meals throughout the day and choosing foods high in protein and complex carbohydrates can help maintain energy levels and prevent muscle wasting.

Mouth sores: Chemotherapy and radiation therapy can cause mouth sores, which can make it painful to eat and drink. Eating soft, moist foods and avoiding spicy or acidic foods may help manage mouth sores.

Dehydration: Colon cancer treatment can cause dehydration, especially if nausea and vomiting are present. Drinking plenty of fluids, such as water, herbal tea, and broth, can help prevent dehydration and promote regular bowel movements.

It is important to discuss any side effects with your healthcare team and work with a registered dietitian to develop a nutrition plan that meets your unique needs and preferences. With the right support, it is possible to manage side effects and maintain good nutrition during colon cancer treatment.

Foods that can help manage treatment side effects

A balanced diet that includes a variety of nutrient-dense foods can help manage the side effects of colon cancer treatment. Here are some foods that may be particularly helpful:

Ginger: Ginger has anti-inflammatory properties and may help reduce nausea and vomiting. Adding fresh or powdered ginger to meals or drinking ginger tea may help manage these symptoms.

Bananas: Bananas are easy to digest and can help manage diarrhea. They are also a good source of potassium, which can be lost through diarrhea.

Oatmeal: Oatmeal is a good source of soluble fiber, which can help prevent constipation. It is also easy to digest and can help manage diarrhea.

Yogurt: Yogurt contains probiotics, which are beneficial bacteria that can help restore the balance of gut bacteria. This can be particularly helpful if antibiotics are used during treatment, which can disrupt the gut microbiome.

High-protein foods: High-protein foods, such as lean meat, poultry, fish, eggs, and legumes, can help maintain muscle mass and prevent muscle wasting. They can also help manage fatigue by providing sustained energy throughout the day.

Green leafy vegetables: Green leafy vegetables, such as spinach, kale, and collard greens, are a good source of fiber, vitamins, and minerals. They may also have anti-inflammatory properties and can help manage inflammation-related side effects.

Berries: Berries, such as blueberries, raspberries, and strawberries, are high in antioxidants and can help manage inflammation-related side effects. They are also a good source of fiber and can help prevent constipation.

Water-rich foods: Water-rich foods, such as cucumbers, melons, and celery, can help prevent dehydration and promote regular bowel movements.

It is important to work with a registered dietitian to develop a personalized nutrition plan that meets your unique needs and preferences. They can help identify foods that may be particularly helpful for managing side effects and provide guidance on how to incorporate them into your diet. They can also provide tips for meal planning and preparation, which can be particularly helpful if fatigue or other side effects make it difficult to cook.

Recipes and meal ideas for during and after treatment

During and after colon cancer treatment, it is important to eat a well-balanced diet that provides the nutrients your body needs to heal and recover. Here are some recipe and meal ideas that can help:

1.Smoothies: Smoothies are an easy and convenient way to pack in a lot of nutrients in one meal. You can combine a variety of fruits, vegetables, and protein sources to create a delicious and nutrient-dense smoothie. Some examples include:

Berry and spinach smoothie: Combine frozen mixed berries,

fresh spinach, Greek yogurt, and almond milk in a blender and blend until smooth.

Tropical smoothie: Combine frozen pineapple, mango, banana, coconut milk, and vanilla protein powder in a blender and blend until smooth.

Green smoothie: Combine fresh kale, banana, peanut butter, and almond milk in a blender and blend until smooth.

2.Soups and stews: Soups and stews are easy to digest and can be a comforting and nourishing meal during and after treatment. Some examples include:

Vegetable and lentil soup: Combine lentils, carrots, celery, onion, garlic, vegetable broth, and spices in a large pot and simmer until the lentils are tender.

Chicken and vegetable stew: Combine diced chicken, carrots, celery, onion, garlic, and chicken broth in a large pot and simmer until the chicken is cooked through and the vegetables are tender.

3.Grilled or baked fish: Fish is a good source of protein and omega-3 fatty acids, which can help reduce inflammation and promote healing. Some examples include:

Grilled salmon: Brush salmon fillets with olive oil and season with salt, pepper, and garlic powder. Grill on high heat for 5-7 minutes per side, or until cooked through.

Baked tilapia: Season tilapia fillets with lemon juice, garlic, and herbs, and bake in the oven at 375°F for 15-20 minutes, or until cooked through.

4.High-protein salads: Salads can be a nutritious and satisfying meal when you add protein sources such as grilled chicken, tofu, or beans. Some examples include:

Greek salad: Combine romaine lettuce, cucumber, tomatoes, red onion, feta cheese, olives, and grilled chicken in a bowl and top with a Greek dressing made with olive oil, lemon juice, garlic, and oregano.

Southwest salad: Combine mixed greens, black beans, corn, avocado, and grilled tofu in a bowl and top with a salsa dressing made with salsa, lime juice, and honey.

It is important to work with a registered dietitian to develop a personalized meal plan that meets your unique needs and preferences. They can provide additional recipe and meal ideas that are tailored to your specific treatment and health status.

CHAPTER SIX

LIFESTYLE CHANGES FOR COLON CANCER PREVENTION AND MANAGEMENT

Beyond diet: *other lifestyle factors that impact colon health*

While diet plays a crucial role in maintaining colon health, there are other lifestyle factors that can also impact your risk of developing colon cancer. Here are some key factors to consider:

Physical activity: Regular exercise can help reduce your risk of developing colon cancer by improving bowel function, reducing inflammation, and lowering insulin levels. Aim for at least 30 minutes of moderate-intensity exercise most days of the week, such as brisk walking, cycling, or swimming.

Weight management: Obesity and carrying excess weight, particularly around the waist, are linked to an increased risk of developing colon cancer. Maintaining a healthy weight through a balanced diet and regular exercise can help lower your risk.

Alcohol consumption: Excessive alcohol consumption has been linked to an increased risk of colon cancer. Limit your alcohol intake to no more than one drink per day for women and two drinks per day for men.

Smoking: Smoking is a known risk factor for many types of cancer, including colon cancer. If you smoke, quit as soon as possible to reduce your risk.

Stress management: Chronic stress can increase inflammation in the body and potentially increase your risk of colon cancer. Find ways to manage stress, such as practicing relaxation techniques, getting enough sleep, and engaging in enjoyable activities.

Screenings: Regular colon cancer screenings can help detect the disease early, when it is most treatable. Talk to your healthcare provider about when you should begin screening and how often you should be screened based on your individual risk factors.

It is important to consider all of these lifestyle factors when it comes to maintaining colon health. Making small changes to your lifestyle can have a significant impact on your overall health and reduce your risk of developing colon cancer.

Exercise and colon health

Regular exercise is one of the most important lifestyle factors for maintaining colon health. Exercise has been shown to help reduce the risk of developing colon cancer, as well as improving outcomes for those who have been diagnosed with the disease.

Here are some of the ways exercise benefits colon health:

Improves bowel function: Exercise helps to stimulate the muscles in the intestines, which can improve bowel function and reduce the risk of constipation. A healthy bowel is important for preventing colon cancer, as it allows waste and toxins to be removed from the body efficiently.

Reduces inflammation: Chronic inflammation in the body has been linked to an increased risk of colon cancer. Exercise has been shown to reduce inflammation in the body, which can help to lower the risk of developing the disease.

Lowers insulin levels: High levels of insulin in the body have been linked to an increased risk of colon cancer. Exercise can help to lower insulin levels, reducing the risk of the disease.

Helps with weight management: Obesity and carrying excess weight are known risk factors for colon cancer. Exercise can help with weight management, which in turn can help to reduce the risk of the disease.

Reduces stress: Chronic stress has been linked to an increased risk of colon cancer. Exercise has been shown to reduce stress and improve mental health, which can help to lower the risk of the disease.

So, how much exercise is enough for colon health? The

American Cancer Society recommends at least 150 minutes of moderate-intensity exercise per week, or 75 minutes of vigorous-intensity exercise per week. Examples of moderate-intensity exercise include brisk walking, cycling, or swimming, while vigorous-intensity exercise may include running or playing sports.

It's important to speak with your healthcare provider before starting a new exercise program, particularly if you have any health conditions or concerns. They can help you develop an exercise plan that is safe and effective for you.

Stress management and colon health

Stress can have a significant impact on overall health, including colon health. Chronic stress has been linked to an increased risk of developing colon cancer, as well as exacerbating symptoms for those who have already been diagnosed with the disease.

Here are some of the ways stress impacts colon health:

Increases inflammation: Chronic stress can lead to increased levels of inflammation in the body, which can contribute to the development of colon cancer. Inflammation in the colon can also exacerbate symptoms for those who have already been diagnosed with the disease.

Impairs digestion: Stress can have a negative impact on digestion, which can lead to constipation, diarrhea, and other gastrointestinal issues. Poor digestion can also contribute to the development of colon cancer.

Weakens immune system: Chronic stress can weaken the immune system, making it more difficult for the body to fight off infections and diseases, including colon cancer.

Impacts lifestyle factors: Stress can also impact lifestyle factors that are important for colon health, such as diet and exercise. For example, when people are stressed, they may be more likely to reach for unhealthy foods or skip their regular exercise routine.

So, what can you do to manage stress and support colon health? Here are some tips:

Practice relaxation techniques: Techniques such as deep breathing, meditation, and yoga can help to reduce stress and promote relaxation.

Exercise regularly: Regular exercise can help to reduce stress and support colon health, as discussed earlier.

Maintain a healthy diet: Eating a healthy, balanced diet can help to support colon health and reduce the risk of developing colon cancer.

Get enough sleep: Adequate sleep is important for overall health and can help to reduce stress levels.

Seek support: Talking to a trusted friend, family member, or healthcare provider can help to alleviate stress and provide support during difficult times.

Managing stress is an important part of overall health and can have a positive impact on colon health. By incorporating stress-reducing techniques and making lifestyle changes, you can support your colon health and reduce the risk of developing colon cancer.

Sleep and colon health

Getting enough quality sleep is important for overall health, including colon health. Studies have shown that lack of sleep can contribute to an increased risk of developing colon cancer, as well as exacerbating symptoms for those who have already been diagnosed with the disease.

Here are some of the ways sleep impacts colon health:

Regulates circadian rhythm: Sleep plays a critical role in regulating the body's circadian rhythm, which is important for many physiological processes, including digestion and immune function. Disruptions to the circadian rhythm, such as those caused by poor sleep, can contribute to the development of colon cancer.

Affects hormone levels: Sleep deprivation can lead to changes in hormone levels, including an increase in stress hormones such as cortisol. Elevated cortisol levels can contribute to inflammation, which is a risk factor for colon cancer.

Impairs immune function: Sleep is important for immune function, and lack of sleep can weaken the immune system, making it more difficult for the body to fight off infections and diseases, including colon cancer.

Contributes to unhealthy lifestyle factors: Poor sleep can contribute to unhealthy lifestyle factors that are important for colon health, such as a poor diet and lack of exercise.

So, what can you do to support colon health through sleep? Here are some tips:

Maintain a regular sleep schedule: Try to go to bed and wake up at the same time each day, even on weekends.

Create a relaxing sleep environment: Keep your bedroom cool, quiet, and dark, and remove electronic devices that emit blue light.

Avoid caffeine and alcohol before bed: Caffeine and alcohol can interfere with sleep quality, so it's best to avoid them before bedtime.

Practice good sleep hygiene: Establish a relaxing bedtime routine, avoid screens before bed, and limit naps during the day.

Address sleep disorders: If you have a sleep disorder such as sleep apnea or insomnia, talk to your healthcare provider about treatment options.

By getting enough quality sleep and making healthy lifestyle choices, you can support your colon health and reduce the risk of developing colon cancer.

8

CHAPTER SEVEN

step-by-step plan to improve diet and lifestyle habits

Making changes to your diet and lifestyle habits can be challenging, but it's important for maintaining colon health and reducing the risk of colon cancer. Here's a step-by-step plan to help you make sustainable changes:

1.Set achievable goals: Start by setting achievable goals that are specific, measurable, and realistic. For example, instead of saying you'll eat a perfect diet every day, set a goal to add one serving of fruits and vegetables to each meal.

2.Keep a food diary: Keeping a food diary can help you become more aware of your eating habits and identify areas where you can make changes. Write down everything you eat and drink, including portion sizes and snacks.

3.Focus on whole foods: Aim to eat a variety of whole foods, including fruits, vegetables, whole grains, lean proteins, and healthy fats. Avoid processed foods and sugary drinks.

4.Increase fiber intake: Incorporate fiber-rich foods into your diet, such as fruits, vegetables, whole grains, beans, and nuts. Gradually increase your intake to avoid digestive discomfort.

5.Drink plenty of water: Staying hydrated is important for overall health, including colon health. Aim to drink at least 8-10 glasses of water per day.

6.Limit alcohol and caffeine: Excessive alcohol and caffeine intake can have negative effects on colon health. Limit alcohol to no more than one drink per day for women and two drinks per day for men, and limit caffeine intake to no more than 400 milligrams per day.

7.Get regular exercise: Exercise is important for colon health and overall health. Aim for at least 30 minutes of moderate exercise most days of the week.

8.Practice stress management: Chronic stress can contribute to inflammation and other negative effects on colon health. Practice stress-reducing techniques such as meditation, deep breathing, or yoga.

9.Get enough sleep: Getting enough quality sleep is important for colon health. Aim for 7-9 hours of sleep per night.

10.Stay accountable: Track your progress and hold yourself accountable. Consider working with a healthcare professional or a registered dietitian for additional support and guidance.

By making these small changes to your diet and lifestyle habits, you can improve your colon health and reduce your risk of developing colon cancer. Remember to be patient with yourself and celebrate your progress along the way.

Meal plans and recipes to support colon health

Meal plans and recipes can be an essential part of a comprehensive plan to support colon health. When planning meals, it is important to consider a variety of nutrient-dense foods that contain fiber, antioxidants, and anti-inflammatory properties. Below are some meal ideas and recipes that can support colon health:

1.Breakfast ideas:
   Greek yogurt with berries and chia seeds
   Oatmeal with sliced banana and almonds
   Spinach and mushroom omelet with whole-grain toast
   Smoothie with spinach, frozen berries, banana, and almond milk

2.Lunch ideas:
   Grilled chicken or salmon with quinoa and roasted vegetables
   Black bean and sweet potato chili with a side salad
   Turkey or veggie burger on a whole-grain bun with avocado and a side of roasted sweet potato wedges
   Greek salad with chicken, feta cheese, and a whole-grain pita

3.Dinner ideas:
   Baked salmon with roasted asparagus and quinoa
   Stir-fry with chicken, vegetables, and brown rice

Lentil soup with a side salad and whole-grain bread
Grilled chicken or tofu kebabs with a side of roasted sweet
potato and broccoli

4.Snack ideas:
  Fresh fruit with nut butter
  Hummus with carrot and celery sticks
  Greek yogurt with berries and granola
  Air-popped popcorn with a sprinkle of nutritional yeast

5.Recipes:
  Quinoa and Black Bean Salad: Cook quinoa according to
package directions. Mix cooked quinoa with black beans, diced
red pepper, diced avocado, chopped cilantro, and a squeeze of
lime juice.

Grilled Chicken with Mango Salsa: Grill chicken breasts until
fully cooked. For the salsa, mix diced mango, diced red onion,
chopped cilantro, and a squeeze of lime juice. Serve the chicken
with the salsa on top.

Roasted Vegetables: Cut up your favorite vegetables (such as
broccoli, sweet potato, carrots, and bell peppers) and toss with
olive oil, salt, and pepper. Roast in the oven at 400°F until
tender.

Green Smoothie: Blend together spinach, frozen berries,
banana, almond milk, and a spoonful of nut butter.
  It is important to note that these meal plans and recipes
are just a starting point. It is essential to tailor your diet
to your individual needs and preferences while considering

your treatment plan and any side effects. Additionally, it is recommended to consult with a registered dietitian or healthcare provider to develop a personalized meal plan.

Tips for staying motivated and making lasting changes

Making changes to your diet and lifestyle can be challenging, especially when faced with the demands of everyday life. However, it is possible to make lasting changes with a few simple strategies. Here are some tips for staying motivated and making lasting changes to support your colon health:

1.Set achievable goals: Start by setting small, achievable goals that are realistic for your lifestyle. For example, aim to eat one extra serving of vegetables per day or to go for a 10-minute walk after dinner. Once you have achieved these goals, gradually increase the difficulty.

2.Keep a food and activity diary: Keeping a diary of what you eat and your physical activity can help you identify areas where you can make improvements. It can also help you stay accountable to yourself and track your progress.

3.Find support: Enlist the support of family, friends, or a health coach to help you stay motivated and hold you accountable.

4.Focus on the positive: Instead of focusing on what you can't eat, focus on the foods that you can enjoy that will support your colon health. Explore new recipes and try new foods to keep things interesting.

5.Prepare ahead of time: Planning and preparing your meals ahead of time can help you make healthier choices and avoid temptation. Set aside time on the weekends to plan your meals and prepare healthy snacks.

6.Make it enjoyable: Incorporate activities that you enjoy into your lifestyle, such as dancing, hiking, or gardening. This can help you stay motivated and make lasting changes.

7.Celebrate your successes: Celebrate your successes, no matter how small they may seem. This can help you stay motivated and build momentum towards achieving your goals.

Here are some meal plan and recipe ideas to support colon health:

Breakfast:

Overnight oats with chia seeds, berries, and nuts
  Scrambled eggs with spinach and whole-grain toast
  Smoothie bowl with Greek yogurt, banana, and berries
  Lunch:

Mixed green salad with grilled chicken, avocado, and quinoa
  Veggie wrap with hummus, roasted vegetables, and feta cheese
  Minestrone soup with whole-grain crackers
  Dinner:

Grilled salmon with roasted Brussels sprouts and sweet potato wedges
  Chicken stir-fry with broccoli, bell peppers, and brown rice
  Lentil soup with whole-grain bread and side salad

Snacks:

Carrot sticks with hummus
Apple slices with almond butter
Greek yogurt with berries and nuts
Remember, making lasting changes to your diet and lifestyle takes time and effort. With patience, persistence, and support, you can achieve your goals and support your colon health.

www.ingramcontent.com/pod-product-compliance
Lightning Source LLC
Chambersburg PA
CBHW051853250726